The Busy Mom's Guide to Healthy *Food* in a Hurry

The Busy Mom's Guide to Healthy *Food* in a Hurry

Enjoy!!
Jennifer L. Beverage

Jennifer Beverage

Copyright © 2015 by Jennifer Beverage
All rights reserved.

ISBN: 1502308258
ISBN 13: 9781502308252
Library of Congress Control Number: 2015901745
CreateSpace Independent Publishing Platform
North Charleston, South Carolina

Dedication

I dedicate this book to my loving husband, Steven who provides unwavering support and encouragement in all my endeavors. I also dedicate this book to my beautiful daughters, Emily and Edynn. You girls inspire me to become a better woman.

With a special thanks to God who put me on this amazing path by giving me the tools I needed in the form of adversity and trials. I know I don't always understand the plan but I am forever grateful I took the leap.

Finally, I would like to acknowledge my illustrator, Lewis James. Thank you for your time and creativity. Your illustrations add the perfect whimsical touch to my book.

Table of Contents

	Introduction ix
Chapter 1	Old Habits Die Hard 1
Chapter 2	New Habits Create a New You 7
Chapter 3	Home Cooking Tips 17
Chapter 4	Grocery Shopping Tips 33
Chapter 5	Reading Food Labels 43
Chapter 6	Organic: To Buy or Not to Buy? 59
Chapter 7	Dining-Out Tips 67
	Conclusion 79

Need More Personalized Attention to Reach
Your Goals? I'd be happy to help! · · · · · · · · · · · 83

Recommended for Further Enlightenment · · 89

Tear-Out Guides for Quick Reference · · · · · · · 91

The Dirty Dozen & The Clean Fifteen · · · · · · · 93

Helpful Quick Reference Shopping Tips · · · · · 95

Introduction

Who exactly is this lady writing a book about *healthy food*? And what would she know about being a *busy mom*? First of all, that lady is me! I'm an Institute for Integrative Nutrition-trained health coach who also happens to have a bachelor of arts degree in psychology. I'm a proud army wife, an Independent Team Beachbody® coach, and the mother of two beautiful daughters. I have gained and lost my share of weight. Oh, and I am a recently converted vegan.

I have been on this journey to health and wellness for as long as I can remember. I grew up in a home amply stocked with chocolate bars, potato chips, boxed convenience foods, and a freezer full of frozen pizzas. Am I making you hungry? We also ate out frequently at McDonald's, Wendy's, and Burger King. But deep down inside, I knew there had to be a better way.

You see, I knew that those "foods," although tasty, were not good for my body. I grew up with a diabetic (Type 2) grandfather who would frequently give himself insulin shots in front of me. Although I didn't fully understand why he had to do that, I had a pretty good idea it had to do with his health and how he was ignoring it. I vowed I would never do that to myself (mainly due to a fear of needles, eek!). This began my nearly twenty-year journey to where I am today.

I don't want you to spend twenty years of your valuable time deciphering all of the nutrition information that is available to you out there. So, in honor of busy moms everywhere, I've written this short and sweet manifesto of food and self-awareness to enable you to feed your family healthy food quick, fast, and in a hurry.

When I talk about food, know that I'm referring to whatever nourishes your mind, body, and spirit. In many cases it is what you put in your mouth but often it has more to do with what you allow and invite into your life. With this in mind, I've included sections relating to the forms of food that feed your mind and spirit, intermixed with the foods that feed your body.

My intention is to make the people in our world healthier. I believe the best way to do that is to teach moms how to take care of themselves and feed their kids well. This, in turn, will affect how the kids feed their future families. It will cause a ripple effect of health and wellness for generations to follow. For today, I choose to start with you and your family. What are you waiting for? Turn the page!

CHAPTER 1
Old Habits Die Hard

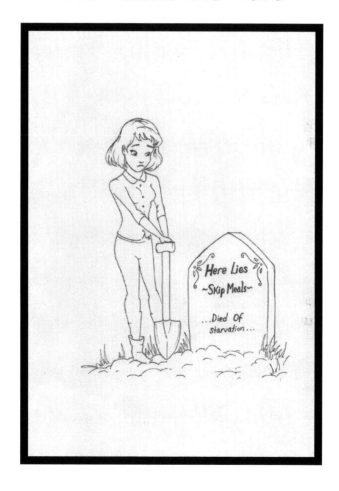

Before I give you helpful tips to feed your family healthy food in a convenient way, let me address some behaviors that won't benefit you, regardless of how healthy your meals are. If you or anyone in your family is skipping meals, using food as a reward, or cutting out entire food groups, stop that immediately! It's also NOT beneficial for you to weigh yourself daily or to play martyr!

Skipping Meals

Just don't do it! Like your car, your body needs fuel. You wouldn't get in your car to drive for three hours with an eighth of a tank of gas, would you? Well, then, why would you start your day without eating breakfast? Skipping a meal doesn't save you calories! It appears to, but trust me, you'll make up for it later.

Our bodies are efficient at keeping the status quo. In other words, they like to maintain balance. If you skip a meal, your metabolism slows to conserve energy. At the same time, your brain reacts to the perceived starvation by telling you to eat everything in sight the next time food becomes available to you. Because of this, you end up eating more calories throughout the day to make up for the meal you missed.

Using Food as a Reward

You've had a long day at work. Little Johnny and Josie drove you nuts all evening with homework, sports, dinner, and baths. They're finally in bed. Time to reward yourself with a hot-fudge brownie sundae, right? Wrong! Don't blow a day's worth of healthy eating and exercise for ten minutes (if that) of ecstasy. This kind of reward feels rewarding only for the short period of time you're eating it. After that, you have the sugar high, followed by the sleepy feeling and brain fog, and then comes the inevitable guilt and self-abuse.

Instead, reward yourself with a hot bath, a good book, or a nice conversation with a friend. Sometimes the treat is more of a coping mechanism than a reward. If this is the case for you, find a positive behavior to replace it with, such as journaling, meditation, or a relaxing walk.

Many parents make the mistake of using food as a reward for their kids. I've been guilty of this, too. Susie won the spelling bee! Let's go out for ice cream sundaes. Bobby scored the winning goal! It's chili-cheese dogs for dinner because they're his favorite.

As parents, we need to teach our children positive behaviors now so that they're not struggling with this as adults. Instead of giving your kiddos sugary, saturated-fat-laden treats, reward them with a trip to the park, a family game night, or a new book.

Cutting Out Food Groups

Let's clear this myth up once and for all: Carbs aren't bad! Now, I feel better, don't you? Carbohydrates are necessary for your body to function properly. You need them! What you don't need is processed junk-food carbs. I'll make it simple: You need carbs from fruits, vegetables, nuts, beans, seeds, and whole grains (brown rice, quinoa, amaranth, millet, oats). You don't need carbs from crackers, cookies, bread, pretzels, chips, tortillas, cakes, pies, and so on. You get the picture.

Cutting out entire food groups robs you of nutrition. You may be thinking, *Wait a minute, didn't she say she was a vegan?* This is a valid point. I cut out meat, dairy, and eggs. Without going into great detail, I put a decent amount of effort into ensuring that I get all the nutrients I need. I am a vegan for ethical reasons, not to cut calories or lose weight (although I have!). As a human being, you need fat, carbohydrates, and protein to function at your best. Taking any one of these nutrients out of your diet is detrimental to your health. Bottom line: Don't do it!

Weighing Yourself Daily or Never

There's nothing more scary or exciting, for a woman trying to lose weight, than stepping on the scale. Some women do it daily and some never, ever, even under threat of tear gas, step on the scale. Both of these extremes are, well, extreme.

Stepping on the scale daily can deliver an unnecessary bruise to your ego. *Why?* You ask. Because your weight fluctuates daily for reasons that have absolutely nothing to do with fat gain or loss! Reasons such as: drinking too much or too little water, eating too much or not enough salt, or hormone fluctuations. There are many other reasons, which are too numerous to list, that cause an inaccurate reading on your scale.

There are some women who choose to never even look at a scale nevermind step on one. I get it. Weighing yourself can be a painful experience, in which you're often left feeling guilty and shameful. I don't blame you for wanting to protect your self-esteem.

The problem is that for many women, this strategy allows the pounds to creep up, year after year. They don't notice just how much they've gained until a shocking photo jolts them into the realization that they have been neglecting their health. Don't let this be you!

I suggest weighing in weekly. Choose one day every week to check in with your health. After all, weight gain or loss can both be predictors of good or poor health. Often weight fluctuations are the first clue a person has that shows up in an obvious way, so please pay attention to it.

The day you choose is completely up to you but I suggest you weigh yourself on the same day every week. I prefer to weigh in on Fridays that way if I slip up on the weekend, I have time to make up for it before my next weigh-in. I also prefer to do it first thing in the morning after my bathroom trip and in the buff (probably TMI but I'm trying to be helpful here). You choose the day and time that works best for you.

Martyring Yourself

As the mother, it's your job to give up on all your hopes and dreams to completely devote yourself to the feeding, teaching, and potty training of your progeny. The second you bring another person into the world, you cease to exist. You live only for the cause. Are you kidding me (insert eye roll here)?

You are not a martyr! You are an amazing woman who was put here on this planet to give your gifts and talents to the world to make it a better place. Raising your kiddos is an important job but it's not your sole purpose for existence. Please know that nurturing and respecting who you are as a person will teach your children to do the same. You deserve to be respected for all you are and all that you do. Accept nothing less.

CHAPTER 2

New Habits Create a New You

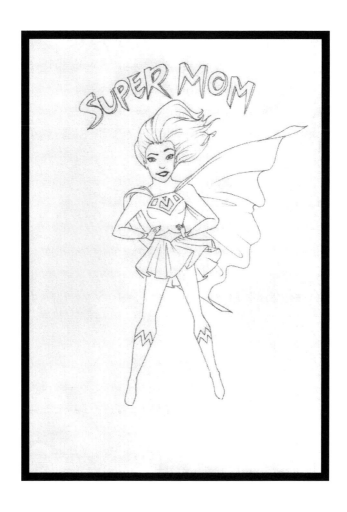

To be the best mother and partner you can be, you need to take care of yourself. Remember, it is never beneficial to you or your family to become a martyr! Self-care takes many forms, depending on what you personally need to feel your best. Some great forms of self-care I recommend are regular exercise, self-beautification treatments, me time, personal development, spirituality, nurturing relationships, and goal-setting.

Exercise

Exercise—you either love it or hate it. There's no in between. I happen to love it, but rest assured, if you're in the other category, you can still make it part of your daily routine. Trust me, it's worth all the benefits you'll receive.

Exercise is good for the body and mind. Of course, we all know the outwardly visible benefits of exercise—a hot bod! As it turns out, it's also good for the mind. Studies have shown that exercise can be as effective as antidepressant meds at altering moods positively (see http://www.health.harvard.edu/newsweek/Exercise-and-Depression-report-excerpt.htm). That means you can sweat for thirty minutes a day, feel great, skip the negative side effects, and save money on a prescription! I don't know about you, but I think that's pretty amazing news.

The benefits are good for your kiddos, too. Regular exercise helps kids focus better, especially when it's time to sit down and learn. And it's good for their bodies. Unfortunately, our bad habits are being passed on to the next generation, and they're feeling the ill effects. Type 2 diabetes used to be known as "adult-onset diabetes," but now it's becoming prevalent in kids. This saddens my heart. Please get your kiddos participating in regular exercise. Go for a family hike or take a walk after dinner every night. Go to the park, have the kids walk the dog, or play tag in your backyard. Do something. Do anything that requires you and your family to move your bodies!

Self-Beautification

Just because you're a mom doesn't mean you don't want to look great or feel good about yourself. You deserve to do things that make you feel pretty. Of course, that means something different to each individual. For some women, it's simply wearing mascara every time they leave the house. For others, it means wearing full make-up, coiffed hair, and fashionable clothing. Still others require coloring their hair, having their nails done, and getting Botox injections.

Wherever you fit on this spectrum is irrelevant. What matters is that you feel pretty and that you do whatever it takes to feel that way. There is a belief that moms who take care of themselves somehow rob their kiddos of something. That's dumb! It's really ridiculous. You can't take care of others effectively if you're neglecting yourself. No ifs, ands, or buts! Anyone who tells you something different is wrong. If they want to argue, please send them my way.

Me Time
Taking time for yourself is crucial to your mental well-being. When I became a mom, I didn't cease being Jennifer the wife, daughter, friend, poet, reader, health enthusiast, runner, writer, student of life, nature lover, and cook. Did you stop being who you were? I hope not, but if you have, now is the time to allow yourself to become you again! I give you permission—even if no one else will.

You deserve to have great joy in your life. While kiddos do bring joy, they're also lots of hard work! Take time daily to do something that's just for you, one thing (or more) that makes your heart sing. Do you love to dance? Then do it! Are you a reading enthusiast? Take time to read each day, even if it's in the bathroom. Does volunteer work feed your soul? Find time to do it and take your kids with you. It's a fantastic learning experience and life lesson for them. Do you want to learn a new language? Go back to college? Learn how to sew, crochet, or knit? Do it! Do it right now! Do it today! I promise you that you will be a better partner, a better mother, and a much more interesting friend!

Personal Development
If you're thinking, *Why is this section labeled 'Personal Development' when clearly all sections in this chapter pertain to it?* You're very observant. In this section, I'm talking about personal development *books*. Never heard of them? You're not alone!

Personal development books should be more appropriately labeled *self-improvement* books. Is there an area you'd like to improve in? Self-confidence? Time management? Organization? Cooking? Interior design? I could literally go on for days because anything and everything you could ever want to improve on, someone wrote the book on it. Guess what? You're reading a personal development book right now. Shut the front door!!!

I read personal development books everyday and it has immeasurably changed my life for the better. Honestly, I can't recommend this enough. I know you don't have lots of time to read and that's okay. Just squeeze in ten to twenty minutes (or more) each day and you will benefit greatly.

Tuck the book, Kindle, Nook, or iPad into your purse or diaper bag and carry it with you throughout your day. I'm guessing there will be times that you're waiting in line for something and can sneak in a few minutes here and there. Spend a lot of time driving? Perfect because personal development books come in audio books too! No money to buy such items? That's okay because your local library will lend them to you for FREE!

There really is no excuse to skip this recommendation. Which books you choose really depend on what you need to work on. I do have one recommended read to get you started: *The Compound Effect* by Darren Hardy. This book has made a positive impact in my life and is suited for any woman who wants to change small daily behaviors in order to yield a large positive impact in her life.

Spirituality

This can be an icky, sticky topic but I'm not easily scared away. Spirituality, you need it. If you don't have it, get it. That's all I have to say about that!

Of course, I have more to say or this would be a very short section in an already short book. When I say spirituality, I'm not referring to religion. They are two distinctly different entities. Spirituality is entirely personal. It is how you relate to your position on this great big rock we call home. Religion generally guides your values and how you choose to practice your beliefs. The two are intertwined for many people but for others they are not. Where you fall on this spectrum makes no difference to me.

What is important is that you have a spiritual practice. This component is key to your happiness and fulfillment in this life. As I said, spirituality is personal. For some it involves going to church weekly and praying daily while for others it involves meditation in nature. Find what makes you feel connected to your purpose, your inner sense of belonging, and your higher self. We are spiritual beings and without connection to our spirits, we feel lost and empty.

If this topic intimidates you and you're not sure where to start, I have a few suggestions. Pick up the Bible, The Torah, The Bhagavad Gita, the Koran or any religious or spiritual text that piques your interest. Start reading and see if it sparks something in you. If that's not your speed start small with anything by Dr. Wayne Dyer. I recommend starting with his book *21 Days to Master Success and Inner Peace.*

Above all, know that there is no wrong answer or wrong way to go about this. Spirituality is intensely personal. Simply follow your heart.

Nurturing Relationships

The world would be a really lonely place without others. For this reason, relationships are an important and necessary part of life. Some relationships bring great joy to your life and others bring great stress. We all want more of the former and less of the latter type of relationships, right? Let's explore how to enrich the quality of all your relationships, whether they're good, bad, or ugly.

First of all, you can't control what others do. Try as you may, it will never work. You can only control you, your thoughts, actions, and behaviors. With this in mind, you need to honor your energy and happiness by minimizing interactions with those who do not honor you and bring only drama and negativity into your life. I know this is difficult in many instances because the negative Nelly is a family member, co-worker, or close friend. Still make every effort to keep contact to a minimum. Your spirit will thank you for it.

When you aren't able to minimize contact, my second tip is to choose kindness. When Aunt Joan is implying that your child-rearing practices aren't up to par with hers and that you're clearly incapable of raising functioning human beings, take a deep breath, remind yourself that she is coming from a place of her own insecurities, and what she's saying has nothing to do with you (hey-it's true! I studied psychology, remember?). Return her criticism with a *Thank you, I never thought of doing it that way*. Then, let it go.

I know this is a huge undertaking but it returns your power where it belongs, with you. It allows you to release her negativity and it takes away her ammunition. I guarantee you, in time, Aunt Joan will stop targeting you. And if she doesn't it won't matter because you won't notice. After all you let go of it a long time ago.

My third and final tip, which will infuse your close relationships with positivity and love, is to give others what you wish they would give you. No, I'm not referring to giving grandma a crisp, hundred-dollar bill because you wouldn't mind finding one in her annual Christmas card. I'm referring to showing others the behavior you'd like to receive from them.

This tip works well with all people you're close to but it works especially well with your spouse or partner. Wish your love would pay more attention to you? Give him more attention. When he's talking to you, instead of staring at your cell phone trolling your Facebook newsfeed and agreeing at the right points in his monologue; make it a dialogue. Look him in the eye while he's talking to you. Engage in what he's saying, even if it doesn't interest you. Genuinely listen to him. We all want to be heard, especially by our partner. Trust me, in time (don't expect it to happen overnight), he will start paying more individual attention to you too.

Do you need more affection from your partner? Start showing him affection. He'll start doing the same to you. Do you want him to help more around the house? Offer him help when you see he needs it and praise him when he offers to help you or does something great without being asked. We all like to be appreciated. Appreciate him more and he'll do more to earn your appreciation.

Goal Setting

Would you get in the car to drive across country without mapping out your journey, packing all the items you'll need, and loading them up in the car (again with the driving analogies!)? No? Well why would you live your life that way?

Unfortunately so many people just go with the flow of life. They never really give much thought to where it will take them. They just roll with the punches and deal with the issues as they come up. That's certainly one way to live life but it's not a very productive way!

If you're one of those zombies, mindlessly walking through life, wake up! Right now! You are here to accomplish great things but those great things will rarely fall into your lap. You have to have a plan. You have to have a purpose. You have to set goals.

Goal setting is fun! Give it a try. Whip out a pen and paper and write down at the top of the page the word

"Goals." Below that word, list what it is you'd like to accomplish. Your goals can be for the next year, the next five years, ten years, or lifetime goals (a.k.a your bucket list). I suggest starting with one-year goals, as it's less intimidating. Once you've listed your one-year goals, break them down into tasks you can do monthly, weekly, and daily to get you to your goal.

If your one year goal is to be debt free, start by adding up all your debt, dividing it by twelve and voilá, you have your monthly payments. Then break it down into weekly goals by dividing it by four and you now know how much money you need to take out of each paycheck to reach your goal. Of course, many goals aren't so easy to break down but I'm trying to get you into the general mindset.

If you find this intimidating, I suggest a personal development book (didn't see that coming, did you?). *PUSH: 30 Days to Turbocharged Habits, a Bangin' Body, and the Life You Deserve!* by Chalene Johnson is a good start. Her book will teach you how to set goals, prioritize which ones to start with, and teach you how to reverse engineer your goal to ensure you know the exact steps you need to take to achieve it. Don't have the time or energy to pick up the book? Head over to www.30daypush.com and Chalene will send you a daily email with videos and tips to get you on the right track! How do I know this works? I know because I've used Chalene's method to reach my goals (hint: your reading the realization of one of my goals right now).

CHAPTER 3
Home Cooking Tips

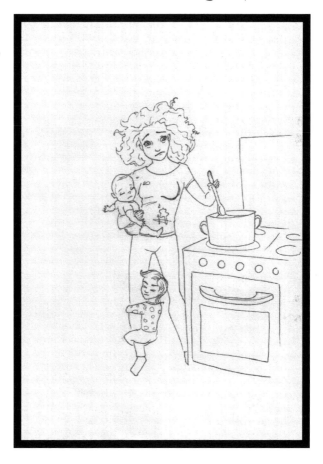

Ah, the joys of home cooking. There's nothing more fun and fulfilling than spending an hour and a half getting dinner on the table, only to have your five-year-old refuse to eat his broccoli or your thirteen-year-old ask in a tone of disgust, *What is this?* Hmm, maybe not so fun or fulfilling.

First of all, unless you're cooking Thanksgiving dinner, there's no need to spend that kind of time in the kitchen. Second of all, your kids will push back when you try to introduce new foods; that's normal. Don't give in and don't be disheartened. Small (and medium) children have little control in their young lives and what they put in their mouths is one of the few things they can control.

I'm here to give you home cooking tips that will help you spend less time in the kitchen, spend less money at the store, save calories, and feel good about what you're putting in your body. Does this sound too good to be true? It's not. It just takes a dash of planning, a sprinkle of know-how, and a pinch of confidence in the kitchen, and voilá! You have more energy, less flab, and optimal health. Let's get started!

To spend less time in the kitchen, you need to take a few key steps: Plan your meals ahead, cook items in batches to be used at more than one meal, double recipes whenever practical, make good friends with your slow cooker, and stock your kitchen with cool gadgets. These steps will ensure that you have healthy food on hand that can be prepared quickly or ahead of time with little effort. Again, I realize this idea sounds too good to be true, but I assure you it is not. I have been using these techniques for years with great success, and I know you can, too. Let's dive into my first tip.

Meal Planning

Planning—not just meals, but anything in life—is your key to success. Do you find yourself making a mental checklist on your drive home from work and wondering if you have enough ingredients to throw together something quick and edible when you get home? Do you end up at the grocery store every day picking something up (and a few extra things—hey, the sale was just too good to pass up!) because you didn't plan your meals or write down everything you would need? Worse yet, are you in the drive-thru of your local fast-food chain three or more times a week because you're tired and you just don't have the time or energy to cook? Stop all of this! It's unnecessary, unfriendly to your budget, unkind to your waistline, and unhealthy for your family. Please remember that the habits you create for your children now will follow them into adulthood and will likely become their life-long habits. From this day forward, I want you to love, honor, and cherish your family's health and feed them food that nourishes them rather than poisons them. Meal planning is easy! You simply have to make time for it.

Starting this week, I want you to sit down on Sunday (really, any day will work; this just seems to be the day most people have spare time) and spend an hour writing out your meal plan. I can hear your shrieks of horror as you're reading this. You're thinking, *I don't have an hour to spare!* Find that hour. Even if you have to get up earlier or stay up later, find the time. It will save you time during the week, not to mention money, extra calories, and poor health! I promise, with practice, meal planning will become second nature, and it won't take an hour out of your week.

Start the process by taking inventory of what you already have on hand in your cupboard, fridge, and freezer. Next, I want you to grab a hot beverage, a pen, a piece of paper, a few favorite cookbooks, and your laptop, and then have a seat in a nice, comfy chair. Now you're going to plan your meals for the week. Knowing what you have on hand will be helpful as you create your grocery list. I want you to browse through your cookbooks and search key words on the Internet until you come up with six or seven meal ideas. Write the meals down in the order you will make them. This is important because you can consider what activities are going on each day and decide which meals will work best on those days. Also be sure to print out online recipes and, if you use a cookbook, note the cookbook name and page number next to each recipe. There's nothing more painful than having to spend time backtracking to find the recipe you planned for tonight's dinner! This also helps you know what you need to put in the fridge to thaw the night before. Keep these meal plans in a handy, dandy notebook or in a document online. You can keep referring back to your favorite meals when you're planning your meals every week. This will save you so much time and effort in the long run! You could even come up with four or five weekly meal plans and rotate them through each month. Below is a sample meal plan for the week:

1. **Meat-Free Monday**:
   Tofu and Veggie Stir-Fry with rice (*Rachel Ray* magazine, p. 75)
2. **Taco Tuesday**:
   Slow-cooked pork tacos with Mexican rice (*Taste of Home* cookbook, p. 121)
3. **Wild-Game Wednesday**:
   Buffalo burgers with homemade sweet potato fries (online, AllRecipes.com)
4. **Try-Something-New Thursday**:
   Tandoori chicken with Indian-style rice, naan bread, and Pav bhaji (SimplyRecipes.com)
5. **Finnicky Friday**:
   Build your own pizza bar
6. **Slack-Off Saturday**:
   Have leftovers or dine out
7. **Succulent Sunday**:
   Pot roast with potatoes and carrots, plus a side salad (*Betty Crocker* cookbook, p. 219)

As you write out your meal plan for each day, look at the recipe and identify which items you already have and which items you need. Immediately write down the items you need on your grocery list and double-check that you have all of the items written down. There is *no* bigger waste of time than having to run to the store two or three times during the week because you forgot to write down an ingredient or two. At first this may feel daunting, but I promise you that if you stick with it for at least a month, it will become nearly effortless, and it will save you *so* much time and energy during your busy weekdays.

Some people choose to plan all of their meals this way, not only dinner, and that's fine. I don't plan other meals; I simply buy breakfast and lunch ingredients to have on hand such as oatmeal, bread, soup, peanut butter, jelly, lunchmeat, cheese, fruit, vegetables and lettuce for salads. For those of you who need healthy ideas for lunches to send to school with your kiddos, I'd be happy to help.

Coming up with delicious, nutritious, and creative lunches (for school or home) for your kiddos every week can be overwhelming. Take heart, it doesn't have to be. First, I'd like you to rethink the typical lunch-box fare. You know the deal: a PB&J sandwich accompanied by Goldfish crackers, fruit snacks, and a Capri Sun. This is not delicious, nutritious, or even remotely creative.

Instead of thinking in terms of filling up their bellies, focus on nourishing their bodies and minds. Pack a wholegrain item, some fruit, some veggies, and a healthy protein. Pack brown rice stir-fry containing carrots, peas, and chicken (any healthy leftovers are great) with an apple. If that doesn't tickle your kiddos fancy, try a finger-food lunch. Pack a mozzarella cheese stick with carrot and celery sticks, ranch dressing (watch out for MSG), grapes, and almonds. Try packing plain Greek yogurt drizzled with honey and topped with fruit and granola accompanied by cucumber slices. Try organic corn tortilla chips with a Mexican dip containing salsa, sour cream, refried beans, and guacamole. Kids always love dipping stuff! If you're not very creative, that's OK. There are lots of great recipes online.

I know you're thinking, *My kid will never eat that in a million years!* You might be surprised. Kids often gravitate toward "kid foods" because that's what we've taught them, not because it's what their little bodies crave. Don't be afraid to think outside of the (lunch) box! Give it a try (or a few). I think you'll be pleasantly surprised.

Cooking in Batches

You've purchased all of the items on your list, now what? Take a look at my menu plan above. Cute names for each day of the week, right? You don't have to do that. It just makes the mundane task more fun and creative! Now down to business. Did you notice that rice is on the menu three times this week? You're quite perceptive. This is not a coincidence. Cooking rice, especially brown rice (which I recommend), can take forever! What you're going to do is save time by cooking a big batch either on Sunday before the week starts or on Monday when you cook the rice for dinner that evening. Then, whenever your menu calls for rice, you simply heat it up and add the prescribed ingredients! I also do this with quinoa (if you haven't tried this ancient grain that's actually a seed, I highly recommend it—*yum*) and beans. This technique works well for lunch items, too. Make a big pot of chicken soup with veggies on Sunday and enjoy it all week long. The same goes for vegetables for salads or snacks. Cut up veggies and put them in containers or bags to grab and go. This tip will help encourage kids (and adults) to eat more vegetables because the hard work has already been done.

Doubling Recipes

This tip seems like a no-brainer but honestly how often do you think to double or triple the amount in a recipe and make three meals instead of one?

Not often enough! Think about how much time you'll save in the weeks to come if you use this strategy. You're already making the recipe once; making more of it won't take nearly as long as making it again in a couple weeks.

This is a win-win strategy because it saves you time, three times! First you save time because you will only be shopping once for the three meals. Next you save time because you'll be preparing the meals at the same time, saving you time in the weeks to come when you would be preparing them. Finally, it saves you time cooking the meals because these only need to be reheated. If you've made a meal that can be cooked or reheated in your slow cooker, even better! This brings me to my next nugget of useful knowledge.

Making Slow-Cooker Meals

I'm willing to bet that you have a slow cooker. I'm also willing to bet that you don't fully understand the joy of cooking when you're not actually in the kitchen cooking! If your slow cooker has been relegated to the back of your cabinet, allow me to persuade you to whip it out and dust it off.

The slow cooker is one of the most used items in my kitchen. I use it at least two or three times a week. Not because I'm too busy to make dinner every night but because there are more interesting things I'd rather be doing! Look back at the meal plan above. Two to three of the items above can be made in the slow cooker depending on the final product you'd like. I highly recommend cooking pork loin or boneless, skinless chicken thighs in the slow cooker at every chance you get! You can cover the meat with BBQ sauce to create BBQ pork sandwiches or cover it with salsa to create chicken tacos. Dump a can of enchilada sauce over the meat and you've got enchilada-filling waiting for you when you're ready to assemble dinner. You just saved twenty to thirty minutes right there! The best part is that I never, ever thaw the meat! I don't even have to plan ahead more than simply having the meat and sauce available. Just place the frozen meat in the slow cooker, cover it with sauce, and cook on the low setting for eight hours or high for four to six hours.

The only caveat I have about this is don't try to place raw (frozen or fresh) ground meat in the slow cooker unless you're itching for *E. coli* or *Salmonella* poisoning. If you've had food poisoning, you know what I'm talking about! It is, however, permissible and even recommended to put cooked, ground meat in your slow cooker for items such as chili, soups, and stews. You're only limited by your imagination. Wait, you have the Internet now, so you're not even limited by that! Simply search Google for "slow cooker recipes" and you could spend days wading through the results you find. I also recommend Googling "freezer slow cooker recipes." These recipes are awesome! You prepare all the ingredients and sauces ahead of time, place them in a zip-top gallon freezer bag, throw the bags in the freezer, and pull them out when you're ready to prepare and enjoy. No thawing necessary. Seriously, it doesn't get any easier than that!

Getting the Most Out of Kitchen Gadgets

The beauty of being born in this day and age is all the gadgetry that has been invented to save time and sanity in the kitchen. There are so many amazing kitchen gadgets that are both fun and helpful. While I'm sure you'd love to read about every, single one of them, nobody's got time for that!

Of course you need to have the basic kitchen gadgets such as: measuring cups (liquid and dry), measuring spoons, spatulas, pots, pans, potholders, knives, can opener, you get the idea. In addition to these necessary items, I'd like to suggest five more gems that will save you time and energy in the kitchen. Of course there are numerous items that will save you time but I'm frugal and prefer items that not only save time but also multi-task. These items include: a flexible cutting board, immersion blender, kitchen shears, microplane, and a food processor.

Cutting boards are a necessary part of any functional kitchen, especially one that turns out healthy food. Flexible cutting boards are particularly useful. Of course, they're great for chopping but they're also great for saving time and keeping messes to a minimum, which again saves more time. In fact, I use my flexible cutting board anytime I'm measuring ingredients for baking. I simply place it underneath the measuring cup or spoon while I pour out the ingredients. When I inevitably spill some, I simply fold the cutting board in half to direct the ingredients and dump the spilled items back into the recipe. The same applies to chopping herbs or veggies for soup or stir-fry. Of course you can do this with a regular cutting board but you better have time, patience, and good aim!

Another handy item to keep in your kitchen is an immersion blender. Now I know that *everyone* has a blender, so why would you need to purchase an immersion blender? Great question! If you're like me, you love warm soups, stews, and chowders when the temps drop. Often times to complete the recipe, you need to blend some or all of the liquid in the pot. If you've tried to transfer hot liquid from the pot to the blender, you know what a hot mess it makes!

The immersion blender makes your job faster and less messy (which equals faster cleanup). Simply stick it in the pot and blend! The great thing about the immersion blender is that it can be used to blend numerous other items such as: sauces, salsa, homemade marinades, smoothies, and pretty much anything you'd use your blender for but with more ease and less cleanup! One caveat though, please beware of sticking your fingers anywhere near the blade. Don't do it! Never, ever! If you feel the need to stick something near the blade to loosen up some gunk, unplug it or remove the battery, and then stick a utensil of some sort down there.

My next suggestion is one of my personal favorites: kitchen shears. I use these all the time and as much as possible. If you've only been taking yours out to cut kitchen twine or packaging, you've been missing out on all the fun! I suggest you use yours to trim meat or cut it into slices for stir-fry; use it to slice herbs; make chopped salad; cut up spaghetti for your kiddos; trim artichokes; chop the rough parts off asparagus; and chop shredded pork for BBQ pork sandwiches. Seriously, I could go on for days here. You're only limited by your imagination (and maybe the sharpness of your shears).

Another invaluable kitchen item is your microplane. If you don't have one, go buy one. Not sure you need one? Read on! Don't you just love chopping garlic and ginger into teeny, tiny, little pieces for recipes? No? That makes two of us. Or maybe hundreds (even thousands) of us depending on how many read this book. The point is: It sucks! The microplane makes this job a breeze. Simply hold the microplane over the pot, pan, or bowl and grate to your heart's content. Other fantastic uses for this awesome gadget include zesting citrus peels, grating fresh nutmeg and cinnamon, or grating parmesan cheese over pasta. All of these foods add a level of deliciousness to your dish that once you've become acquainted with you won't want to live without!

My final recommendation for awesome, time-saving, kitchen gadgets is (drum roll, please) a food processor. I'm ashamed to admit that I've had one of these for years but only started using it in the past year. When I think of the time I wasted not taking advantage of all the nutritious deliciousness I could've been imparting to my family, I just hang my head. A food processor saves you so much time shredding, chopping, and slicing. It also does the mixing too. Did you know that you can make pesto, salsa, homemade nut butters, mayo, dough for pasta, pizza, or bread too? There's so much more you can make with this invaluable gadget. If you have one that you've been ignoring, please pull it out, apologize, search Google for "food processor recipes" and get reacquainted.

Entertaining

Sometimes you feed more than your family, a.k.a entertaining. I don't know about you but I don't enjoy *entertaining* when I'm stuck in the kitchen not actually interacting with the people I'm supposed to be entertaining. It's not a coincidence that I've saved entertaining for the last part of this section. All the other suggestions I've detailed in this chapter, in conjunction with an additional important tip, will help make entertaining fun and easy.

The most important tip to entertain with ease is to plan meals that you can make the majority of the items ahead. Cut veggies and fruit ahead of time. Assemble casseroles or other items ahead and refrigerate them. Make sauces, dips, and spreads beforehand. Anything you can do the day or even many hours before the party, do it! This will save you so much time and stress before the party. You won't be frazzled when guests arrive and you may even enjoy yourself at your own party.

I mentioned above that all the tips in the chapter are helpful for party planning but some are more useful and I'd like to highlight a couple of those now. First, use your slow cooker for parties. Trust me, it's like having another chef in the kitchen. Cook soups, stews, chowders, roasts, BBQ ribs, veggies, casseroles, or anything your heart desires in this one pot wonder! While it's playing head chef, you can be sous chef and chop any last minute items you'll need for the meal such as herbs, veggies, or salad stuff. Heck, throw caution to the wind and purchase a second slow cooker to use for such occasions! Trust me, it'll be worth it.

The second tip, which I mentioned in a previous section, is to make one item and use it many times in many dishes. Cook hard-boiled eggs and make deviled eggs, put chopped eggs in your potato salad, and serve sliced eggs on your salad bar. This works well with rice too. Serve Mexican fiesta rice with your taco bar, use rice in your chicken enchilada soup, and serve Mexican rice pudding (arroz con leche) for dessert. Cook the rice once and use it three times to get the maximum benefit for minimum effort.

CHAPTER 4
Grocery Shopping Tips

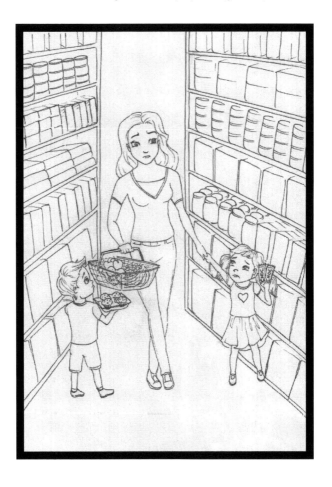

Now that you have your grocery list in hand, whether it's to feed your family or entertain, let's take on the grocery store. Ah, the dreaded supermarket filled with oh, so many choices. Seriously, like six hundred fifty thousand products to choose from! Because of this, each trip is sure to leave you mystified and scratching your head for at least an hour every week. How do you navigate the grocery store so that you arrive home with only nutritious and delicious, whole foods for your family, while avoiding the dreaded chemicals, additives, and preservatives? Great question! Let me show you how to navigate the grocery store with ease and avoid the many, many processed-food traps.

Hunger Trap

This trap can be the most detrimental to your waistline and your budget! Never, I repeat, NEVER go grocery shopping when you're hungry! Grocery stores thrive on this sort of unpreparedness. Next time you're in the store, look around at all the signs with delicious food on them, take a big whiff of the scrumptious smells wafting from the deli and bakery areas, and look at the food packages themselves. These are all ploys to get you to buy more. If you're not hungry, you can reason your way out of this trap but if you're tummy is rumbling, forget it. You can add twenty percent to your grocery bill and a few pounds to your waistline. If you'd like to avoid either of those fates, there are a few tips I can share to keep you from falling victim to this trap.

GROCERY SHOPPING TIPS

Whenever possible, go shopping directly after you've had a meal. This will keep you focused on the task at hand and keep your mind (and feet) from wandering to the bakery. If shopping isn't practical immediately after eating, take heart there's a simple trick to keep you from shopping on an empty stomach. I suggest you keep healthy snack food on you at all times. Keep fresh or dried fruit, nuts, seeds, granola, or whole food bars (such as Kashi bars or Trio bars) in your coat, purse, or car for such emergencies. While you're at it keep some water with you too. Sometimes we mistake thirst for hunger and this will keep you well hydrated. Try to eat your snack and drink the water before arriving at the supermarket to give your tummy time to tell your brain it's satiated. Once you're feeling in control of your stomach, head into the store.

Flyer Trap

Every Sunday and oftentimes during the week the local grocery stores are kind enough to send out a flyer. They just want to aid you in planning your weekly shopping trip. They're so darned helpful!

While I agree that the flyers can be useful tools in planning what items you'll buy each week, they can also be seductive temptresses of sale. What I mean by this is that grocery stores are smart and they employ psychology to get you into their stores. They put the best deals on the front page of their ads to get you to shop with them. They're actually willing to take a loss on certain items just to win your trust and your favor. This tactic is called "loss leader advertising." Once you're in the store purchasing the inexpensive item you're more likely to purchase other items that they sample or put on endcaps or mid-aisle displays. More about those later.

To avoid this tactic, be smart and savvy about where you shop. Many stores price match now so use this to your advantage (look up their price matching policy before visiting the store). Gather all the flyers up, circle all the great deals, and choose one of the price matching stores to cash in on your thriftiness. If this isn't an option, as some local grocery stores don't price match, decide if it's worth saving a couple pennies to drive to two plus stores to get all your items. If all else fails, simply choose the store with the most sales that interest you and shop there!

Coupon Trap

Anyone who has ever set foot inside of a supermarket knows that there are numerous processed-food traps. Before you even get in the store, items such as flyers and coupons tempt you to purchase unhealthy items. How often have you encountered a coupon for fresh broccoli, apples, or avocados? Not often, I'm sure. Do you know why? It's because broccoli farmers don't have the money to offer coupons. Their profits are minimal. Big food companies that use inexpensive commodity crops (corn, soy, wheat) in their food, on the other hand, can afford to save you twenty-five cents on their taco shells or potato chips. If you take away nothing else from this book, please remember this: You get what you pay for! This is true in every area of your life, but it is especially true about food. The typical Sunday paper coupons will save you money now, but trust me, you will pay for it later. Coupons aren't inherently evil. The problem is they get well-meaning, intelligent adults to buy unhealthy food items they otherwise wouldn't even consider, simply because they can save money.

To avoid the *coupon trap* and shop smart you need to learn to use coupons to your advantage. Most people look in the Sunday paper and clip whichever coupons tickle their fancy. I suggest you seek out the coupons you need to create the nutritious meals you want to prepare for your family, instead of simply hoping to come across them. How do you do this? Use the Internet, of course! Google "use coupons to eat healthy food" and you will instantly have 24.8 million results at your finger-tips. If that's not efficiency, then I don't know what is. Since neither you nor I have the time to sift through that many results, I suggest checking out the first five or ten websites that appear on the page. There you will be given great tips on where to find and how to use coupons to buy foods that are actually good for you and your family.

Endcap Trap

Coupons aren't the only ploy used to tempt you away from your good intentions. Ever notice the endcap and midaisle displays? The foods on them are meant to tempt you into buying what you didn't know you wanted or needed! Avoid these at all costs. How often do you see an endcap or display with produce? Rarely. And you never see this anywhere in the store other than the produce aisle. How often do you find S'mores items or other baking ingredients in a cleverly designed aisle display in the produce section? Frequently! Just walk right past these flagrant displays of trickery. Ignore the pretty colors and signs offering low prices. Remember, you get what you pay for!

A good rule of thumb is: if it's not on your list don't purchase it! This will keep you from falling victim to temptation. Sometimes you actually do need the item on display. While I'm certain this is the exception rather than the rule, you must decide for yourself. Distinguish between a need and a want. Not sure how? Is this an item necessary for an actual meal? Will this item nourish your kiddos or only fill their bellies? Would it generally be considered a treat or dessert item? If it's not something vitally necessary to making breakfast, lunch, or dinner and isn't made solely by Mother Nature, skip it.

Sample Trap

Another in-store attempt to derail your good intentions is food samples. You go into the store to pick up milk and bread and walk out with three more items because you decided to sample a cheese ball, and now you must buy the ingredients required for it in the hope of having an occasion to make a cheese ball in the near future. Do not let this be you! How often are those samples real, whole foods?

The answer is almost never. If they are whole foods such as broccoli or carrots, they're sure to be accompanied by ranch dressing or some other unhealthy dip or sauce. Just keep walking. I know it feels like you're getting something for free, but it's more cleverly disguised trickery!

This trickery plays on the social standard known as the rule (or norm) of reciprocity. The vendor is giving you something for free in hopes that you will feel obligated to purchase something in return. Keep this psycho-babble in mind next time you're feeling guilty for sampling the cheese ball and crackers without purchasing. You may just leave the store with lighter bags and a fuller bank account.

Superstore Trap

I'm not going to lie; I'm a fan of Superstores. There I said it! Where else can you pick up ingredients for dinner, a birthday card for grandma, thread to mend hubby's socks, dog treats for Fido, and yoga pants all in one very large room? Nowhere! Superstores are great time-savers but if you're not careful they're also a great place to empty your wallet.

This is a place where good intentions go south quickly. Use your judgment and refer to the tip above. Do you need the $5 DVD or do you want it? Do you really need a pumpkin scented candle, Barry Manilow's greatest hits CD, Easter bunny socks, or a t-shirt that reads "I'm not short I'm fun-sized"? Probably not! Keep your wits about you, stick to your list, and you'll make it out with your budget intact.

Shop the Real-Food Aisles

The best advice I have to give is to stick to the produce section and the outer aisles of the grocery store. You may have heard this before, but I'm repeating it because it's useful advice. Where do you get most of the items that go in your shopping cart? Next time you're in the grocery store, consider that question. Look at others' carts and see where they get most of their items.

I frequently look in others' carts wondering what they put into their bodies for fuel. Recently on a shopping trip to the local grocery store, I was food-peeping and decided to look up. Guess who I saw predominantly in the produce aisles? The elderly. Guess why they're there? If you're thinking *Alive or in the produce section?* The answer is both! They're enjoying longevity *because* they shop mainly in the produce section.

Generally this section is located in the front of the store. You should spend most of your time and money in the produce section. The best part is that you don't have to read labels. Everything in this section that is label-free is good for you! The only choice you need to make is whether to buy organic or not. I go into depth about that subject in a future chapter.

Other parts of the store that are relatively safe are the meat and dairy sections and some *parts* of the frozen-food aisle. This area of the store is a little bit tricky because you have to read labels. I will teach you how to read food labels in an upcoming chapter. Pay attention

GROCERY SHOPPING TIPS

to the quality of the items you're buying. Look for the smallest number of ingredients on the label and make sure they sound more like food than a chemistry experiment that you performed in high school. If you're buying meat, shouldn't the label read only "chicken" or "beef"? If you're buying cheese, milk should be the first ingredient. As a side note, please run far away from bright-orange cheese-like substances. There is no nutritional or redeeming value to these items. Once you start eating real, whole foods, I promise you that you will no longer enjoy the taste of such food-like substances.

In the frozen-food aisle, look for the item you're purchasing (broccoli, strawberries, spinach) to be the first and preferably the only ingredient on the label. Stick to purchasing mainly frozen fruits, vegetables, and meat in the freezer section of the store. Don't buy frozen lasagna or enchiladas. Make them yourself. This will give you the peace of mind to know there aren't any hidden chemicals or food additives in your meal.

CHAPTER 5

Reading Food Labels

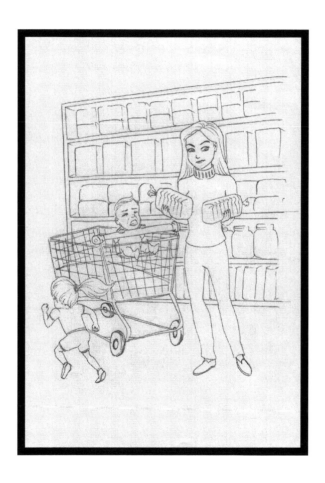

Now that you've learned how to navigate the various pitfalls of the supermarket, let's go into depth about one of the most important tactics in the war against putting chemicals and food-like substances into our bodies: label reading! This section is a labor of love for me. I am an avid label reader. I have, on occasion, spent twenty minutes in the bread aisle deciphering labels to decide which item would provide the most nutrition and do the least amount of harm to my family. So you won't need to do this, I'm going to share my tips and secrets with you. After reading this section, you'll know what to look for on ingredient labels, what to avoid, and how to understand nutrition facts.

Less Is More

First and foremost, less is more! Less, or fewer, ingredients, that is. The fewer ingredients there are in an item, the closer it is to the food God intended. When buying anything that comes in a package (a.k.a. processed food), I aim for three to five ingredients at most. Take peanut butter, for example. Many peanut butter labels read "natural" on the front, but a quick turn of the jar reveals that it's not even close to being natural. The claim "natural" is not regulated by the FDA at this point, so any company can put it on any product with the hope that a well-intentioned consumer doesn't turn the package around. Call me old-fashioned, but I prefer my peanut butter to consist solely of peanuts! No added sugar, salt, or palm oil—just delicious and nutritious peanuts. The best part is that nearly every grocery store sells real peanut butter without any additives or preservatives. This brings me to my next point.

Food Additives and Preservatives

Additives and preservatives are bad news! Common food additives and preservatives include: artificial coloring, sodium benzoate, high-fructose corn syrup, trans fat, monosodium glutamate, aspartame, and sodium nitrate. Let's look at each additive individually. For further reference, I found the following information about additives and preservatives on the webmd.com website at http://www.webmd.com/diet/features/the-truth-about-seven-common-food-additives.

First we have artificial coloring. The stuff that makes cheese puffs an obnoxious bright orange color is not found in nature! It seems harmless enough and makes our food oh, so colorful. There are conflicting studies, so the jury is still out, but some food coloring has been linked to hyperactivity in kiddos and asthma in individuals of all ages. I don't know about you, but that's reason enough for me to avoid giving it to my children. Here is a list of FDA-approved colorings and their common names as listed on ingredient labels:

- FD&C Blue No. 1 (brilliant blue FCF)
- FD&C Blue No. 2 (indigotine)
- FD&C Green No. 3 (fast green FCF)

- FD&C Red No. 40 (allura red AC)
- FD&C Red No. 3 (erythrosine)
- FD&C Yellow No. 5 (tartrazine)
- FD&C Yellow No. 6 (sunset yellow)
- Orange B (hot dog and sausage casings)

I have had personal experience with the effects of food coloring. I love peanuts enrobed in milk chocolate covered with a colorful, candy-coated shell! During a past move with the army, this item was my comfort food of choice. In the evening, when I was feeling exhausted from the day, I would comfort myself with a bag of peanut-filled chocolate candies. After about five days of doing this, I became very depressed, unlike I had felt in a long time. Because of research I had done, I was aware of the possible mood-altering effects of food coloring, and I started to wonder if there was a connection. So I stopped eating the candy and within twenty-four hours, the depression was gone and didn't return! Is it possibly a coincidence? I suppose it's possible. I share this with you in case you struggle with depression or anxiety. Tweaking your diet to remove excess and unnecessary additives could repair and improve your quality of life.

Next, let's talk about sodium benzoate. I know it sounds like something that belongs in a science lab, but it is found in your food! This additive is used to preserve foods and prevent molding. Sodium benzoate is typically found in such items as soda, fruit juice, and salad dressings. It has been shown to increase hyperactivity in children as well. Hmm, I wonder if the increase in consumption of processed foods has anything to do with the increase in ADHD in kids? Just some food for thought (wink, wink).

On down the line, we have high-fructose corn syrup. Ah, my arch nemesis! This additive is found in *everything*! It's made from corn, and it's cheaper than sugar, so naturally food companies use it in sugar's place. If you like increasing and storing body fat, by all means eat this ingredient in abundance. But if you prefer a trim and healthy body, avoid this ingredient. Right now you're thinking, *I don't consume large amounts of high-fructose corn syrup because I have only an occasional soda.* Think again. Unless you're making a conscious effort to avoid it, you're getting a healthy daily dose of it in your ketchup, barbecue sauce, bread, etc. Please, please, please read labels. This insidious ingredient is hidden everywhere, and it's causing Americans to become obese, diabetic, and generally unhealthy.

Next up is trans fat. I'm sure you've heard about this one because it has come under fire in recent years, and for good reason. Trans fats are an unnatural product formed by adding hydrogen to oil. Our bodies don't know how to process these fats, so they just store them—in our arteries! This additive has no place in your diet.

Trans fats are required to be listed in the Nutrition Facts section. Please be thorough and also read the ingredients because if there is less than a certain amount in the product, it can be listed as 0 g of trans fat per serving. Upon reading the ingredient label, you may notice that it says "hydrogenated oil" or "partially hydrogenated oil." Those are trans fats, and you need to steer clear of that product. Remember if you're getting a little trans fat here and a little there, that will add up and negatively affect your body.

Next in the line of fire is monosodium glutamate, famously found in Chinese food. The truth about this additive is that we don't have studies supporting the notion that it's not good for us. Some people have a sensitivity to it, but it's believed to be rare. I, personally, try to avoid it because why take the chance? I have to admit, though, this isn't an easy one to avoid in our house because my kids are avid ranch-dressing eaters, and it's found in nearly *every* brand! Decide what's right for you and your family.

Now we come to aspartame. Another enemy of mine! I'm not going to lie; I used to drink diet soda frequently. A sweet carbonated drink with no calories—what's not to love? Um, if something has flavor, shouldn't it have calories? I think so now. In fact, you couldn't pay me to drink a diet soda! I avoid artificial sweeteners with a vengeance. Even sucralose, my long-time go-to calorie-free sweetener. The truth is, these are chemicals that mess with your body. From the moment the sweet treat hits your tongue, it causes the same response in your body that sugar does. Your body releases insulin to move the sugar in your blood to your organs to provide nutrients, except no sugar arrives. This increased insulin in your body causes your blood sugar to drop dramatically, which causes you to crave—guess what—*sugar*! Next thing you know, you're craving carbs like it's nobody's business, and you're feeling tired and lethargic. Skip the drama! If you have to have a soda, drink the real thing on rare occasions or try sweetening carbonated water with a splash of real fruit juice.

Finally, we have sodium nitrate. This gem of an additive is found in many processed meats such as hot dogs, sausages, and lunchmeat. Americans were having issues with increased gastric cancer before refrigeration came along and took away the necessity to cure all our meats. Now that we eat less cured meat, there is less incidence of gastric cancer. The takeaway is don't eat processed, cured meats on a regular basis. If you're making salami sandwiches for your kids' lunch and you're feeding them a hot dog or sausage at dinner, you may want to rethink what ingredients are in the items you're feeding your family. While you're rethinking the ingredients, take a moment to learn the alternate names for various ingredients you may want to avoid.

Alternative Names for Common Ingredients

If you or anyone in your family has food allergies then you know how hard it can be to figure out what ingredients some items really have in them. Fortunately common allergens such as wheat, milk, eggs, soy, and nuts are listed on food labels in bold print underneath the ingredients list. Unfortunately other ingredients that are allergens or foods you'd like to avoid are listed more stealthily. I can't eat anything with corn in any form in it unless I want gas, bloating, or stomach cramps. Corn isn't listed as a common food allergen so I have to do my research. Many times corn is listed plainly as corn syrup, cornstarch, or corn flour but sometimes it shows up in the form of modified food starch, maltodextrin, or many other unclear terms. This makes it hard to really know what you're eating. This is all the more reason to eat items with fewer ingredients or whole foods with no label at all.

Of course I know this isn't always practical so I want you to be armed with the knowledge that will help you determine what you're actually eating. Did you know a quick Google search reveals fifty plus names for sugar on ingredient labels? Because of this, I could write a whole (boring) book on alternative names for sugar, wheat, corn, soy, or dairy. Instead of taking up too much space in this (interesting) book, I added this section to make you aware that ingredients aren't always what they seem. When in doubt, look it up by searching Google for "other names for ingredients" and you'll find numerous sites dedicated to helping you decipher product ingredients. Isn't technology nifty?

As you know, ingredients aren't the only information listed on product labels. You'll also find nutrition claims and nutrition facts! Let's explore the enigma of nutrition claims now.

Nutrition Claims

Just because the label on the box claims the item is healthy, it doesn't mean it's actually good for your body. Who puts the nutrition claim on the box? The company who will make money from you purchasing it! Do you suppose they have a motive other than your health? I know they do. For this reason, I want you to scrutinize every health claim you encounter. If they have to dress the item up as healthy, chances are you shouldn't eat it!

The most prevalent health claim that is just ridiculous to me is the term "natural." Natural means made in nature, by Mother Earth, not by man. Yet they slap this label on everything. I've seen the word "natural" on packaging for potato chips, cheese puffs, French fries, ice cream, pet food and even soda. It's down right ludicrous! Have you ever seen a soda bush? How about an ice cream tree? No? Me either.

Fortunately this claim has come under much deserved scrutiny and will start to be regulated in the near future. The point I'm trying to make is don't believe what you read. Question it! If it says natural then there should only be one ingredient in it and it doesn't need a package!

Another claim that had me fooled for years is "whole grain." We should all eat more whole grains, right? They have more fiber, more protein, and less impact on your blood sugar. This is all true if you're actually referring to whole grains, not whole grain bread, pasta, boxed breakfast cereals (even ones with heart health claims on them), tortillas, or any baked goods (even bran muffins).

Whole grain means the whole grain is intact. This includes items such as quinoa, millet, amaranth, brown rice, oats (not the processed kind in the convenient packets), farro, barley, etc. These are grains that are good for you. Do not get confused and start buying "whole grain" flours made of these grains, they're not any better for you (okay maybe slightly but not much). If the grain has been processed into anything other than the actual grain, it will not increase your health.

To further clear this up, I'll describe the difference between whole-wheat flour and white flour. This should help you understand it better and allow you to make an educated decision. Whole-wheat flour is made when the whole-wheat grain is pulverized into flour. White flour is pulverized into flour after the outer hull of the wheat is removed. So while the whole wheat flour provides some extra protein and fiber, it essentially has the same impact on your blood sugar; it increases it quickly. Anything that causes your blood sugar to spike causes you to store fat, not to mention a whole slew of other ill health effects.

"Sugar-free" is another claim that has my knickers in a twist! When they take the sugar out, they put artificial sweeteners in sugar's place. Bad, bad, and very bad! Artificial sweeteners have no place in anyone's diet. No, not even diabetics. They are chemical concoctions that are toxic to our bodies. Instead of eating sugar-free items, start eating real, whole foods that are made with sugar, such as fruit, which also conveniently contain fiber (helps to lessen the blood sugar spike). Accompany the fruit with some nuts to help further diminish the impact of the sugar on your body.

Once you cut out the added and artificial sweeteners, you will find naturally sweetened foods very satisfying.

A claim that has been popularized by diet fads is "low carb." The idea is that when you cut back on carbs, you loose weight effortlessly (if you can call physically restraining yourself from eating delicious Italian bread effortless). The problem with this (and all diet fads) is that it was taken to the extreme. For some strange reason fruits and vegetables got lumped in with pizza, bread, pasta, and cookies. Can you see the ridiculousness in this train of thought? Carbohydrates aren't bad. Our body needs them to function well. Processed carbohydrates are bad. They always will be.

To supply the public with the low carb foods we demanded, the food manufacturers did us the favor of making processed junk, low carb! Ugh, when will we get off the diet roller coaster the popular media and food companies have us on, listen to our bodies, and eat real food? Sorry I digress. "Low carb" foods that are processed aren't good for you. They won't help you lose weight in a meaningful and lasting way and they don't even taste good! My advice, forget it.

While we're on the subject of fad diets manipulated by the food industry (and diet participants) let me just say a little about the Paleo diet. At face value, the Paleo diet is great because it gets rid of the excess sugar and focuses on real, whole foods. Awesome! The problem is the diet parameters are being stretched to include baked goods with coconut or almond flour. Umm, don't let me be the bearer of bad news but it misses the point! Flour in anyone form isn't healthful for your body. I apologize if I've burst your bubble but I want you to be equipped with all the information necessary to make healthful diet choices for you and your family.

Finally, I come to the "low fat" claim. I'll make this simple. Fat isn't bad for you. Fats that have been played with by food chemists wearing lab coats are bad for you a.k.a trans fats or hydrogenated oils. Your body needs fat to survive. What do they add to foods after they take out the fat to make them palatable? Naturally fat free sugar, of course. Bottom line, fat doesn't make you fat. Processed sugar does. Any questions? No. Great, let's move on to good ol' nutrition facts.

Nutrition Facts

If you've ever been on a diet, I'm sure you're familiar with the "Nutrition Facts" section of packaged food items. What you may not know is that there is more information than just calories, carbohydrates, and fat content on there! Who knew? Let's start from the top of the standardized "Nutrition Facts" label and work our way down.

First you have the "serving size." This tidbit of information is *really* important. Many small packages that appear to contain one serving actually have more. You know those king-size boxes of M&M's you get at the movie theater? Do you share them with another 1.5 people? I know I didn't,

READING FOOD LABELS

but they contain 2.5 servings. Do you share your twenty-ounce soft drink that you purchase at the gas station with someone else? Probably not, but it also contains more than one serving. Please be mindful of how many servings you're making/consuming. When you're making pasta for a family of four, do you make the whole box and then divide it into four equal portions? Did you know that most boxes have about seven servings of pasta in them? This brings me to the next section.

Under serving size, you find "servings per container." This information is especially helpful when using recipes. If the recipe calls for four cups of chicken stock, you can do some quick math. Multiply the serving size by servings in the container to find out if one box will be enough. This information is also helpful when making yourself feel bad after eating a whole package of Oreos. *Wow, I ate eighteen servings, which is thirty-six cookies!* I suggest taking one serving out of the bag and then putting the bag somewhere really hard to get to so that you're not tempted to eat more or at least if you are you have to burn a few extra calories climbing shelves or crawling through the crawl-space in the garage to retrieve the bag!

You also will see the amount of calories, total fat, cholesterol, sodium, total carbohydrate, and protein per serving. This is the "meat and potatoes" of the Nutrition Facts. You'll pay attention to the areas you're concerned with. For example, if you're on a diet, you may be more interested in the calories and total fat sections than the sodium or cholesterol sections. If you have high blood pressure, the sodium section will be important to you. If you're counting carbs, avoiding sugar, or trying to get more fiber into your diet, the total carbohydrate section will be of particular interest to you. If you have cardiovascular issues, the cholesterol and total fat sections will be most pertinent. Finally, if you want to build muscle, the protein section will be where you look.

The truth is that no section is more important than any other. They all paint an overall picture of the healthfulness of the product. Honestly, I don't pay much attention to the calories or total fat information anymore because fat is not the enemy, and it's not as simple as calories eaten versus calories burned. I want fiber and protein in my food because fiber cleans my system out and protein builds my strong muscles. I don't want excess sugar, cholesterol, or saturated fat because those items will cause diabetes, inflammation, and heart disease. Finally, I don't want more than three to five ingredients because the closer the item is to the way God made it, the better it is for my body. Of course, there are special occasions when you simply want a Twinkie, but they should be rare occasions, and such foods should not be part of your regular diet.

I know you're sitting there thinking, *Great! Now what am I supposed to eat?* The answer is simple! Eat real, whole foods. The foods your grandparents ate as kids. The type of foods that don't come with a label. Eat fresh, grass-fed beef and free-range chicken. Eat lots of fruits, vegetables, raw nuts, and seeds. Eat beans, rice, quinoa, and oats. If your diet consisted of mainly these ingredients, as generations before did, you and your family would be in optimum health. You would likely avoid obesity, diabetes, heart disease, high blood pressure, high cholesterol, and cancer.

The change starts with you. You have the opportunity to change the way your family eats, which in turn will change the way your kids feed their families and perpetuate good health through the generations. You can do that! Start today. I promise that you won't regret it, and you'll look and feel better than you have in years!

CHAPTER 6
Organic: To Buy or Not to Buy?

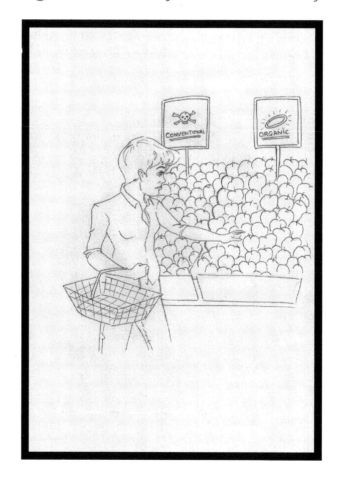

Organic: to buy or not to buy? That is the question! There are a couple key differences between organic and nonorganic items. Organic produce is grown without synthetic pesticides; organic crops are not genetically modified; organic, packaged items have higher-quality ingredients; and organic food tends to cost more than conventional food. I think these differences are worth considering. Hopefully after reading this section, you will, too.

Organic Defined

You may have noticed, during one of your many jaunts to the grocery store, there are different designations for organic foods. If you are confused by the differences, have no fear, I've been sent here to enlighten you! I want to ensure that you fully understand what you're putting in your cart and eventually your body, so I will clarify what each of the terms mean.

"100 percent Organic" means that every ingredient in the item is organic. The terms "USDA Organic" or "Certified Organic" means that 95 percent of the ingredients are organically sourced with the rest coming from ingredients held to a higher standard. "Made with organic ingredients" means that a minimum of 70 percent of the ingredients are organic and the other 30 percent have to follow certain higher standards as well. If you'd like more information about organic regulations check out the www.ams.usda.gov website.

One of the benefits of purchasing items with these designations is less pesticide going into your little one's bodies. Another important benefit is higher quality ingredients that you can actually recognize and pronounce. Unfortunately one of the drawbacks is these items tend to be more expensive. When you're considering whether to buy organic or not, remember you get what you pay for.

Pesticides

Now let's talk about pesticides. Synthetic pesticides are toxic to insects and are used on everything that is grown conventionally. Of course, proponents of pesticides would say that each item contains only a small amount of residue, which can be washed off easily before eating. Let's think about this for a minute. How can pesticide residue be washed off easily? Plants require water to grow. The water sitting on the outside of the plant doesn't make it grow; absorbing the water does. Doesn't it seem likely that the plant is also absorbing the pesticides sprayed onto it? Of course it does! So if each conventionally grown item (wheat, corn, fruits, vegetables, beans, etc.) you ingest has a little bit of pesticide toxins in it or on it, doesn't that add up to a lot of pesticides in your body on a daily basis?

Because your body doesn't recognize the pesticides as food, it can't process and eliminate them. Instead it stores these toxins in your body fat. This means that the toxins don't go away! They just hang around, poisoning your body.

Because human beings start eating at around five months of age (please don't think for a second that baby foods don't have pesticides in them) and live into their seventies and beyond, that's a lot of time to be collecting toxins and suffering the ill effects (often in the form of various cancers). What does a person do to remedy this situation? There are a few options.

Buy organic whenever possible. Not all items are available organic in the supermarket, and some are available only at certain times of the year. Get them when they're available and buy organic as often as you can. If you're on a tight budget and have only a little wiggle room, spend the extra money to purchase the organic counterpart of the conventionally grown items that tend to have the most pesticides on them. These are known as the "dirty dozen." Please refer to the Environmental Working Group's website, ewg.org, for a complete list (or see the convenient tear-out guide in the back of this book).

Another alternative to spending more on organic is to grow your own food. I know not everyone lives on a farm with sprawling fields. You don't need to. In fact, all you need is a small slab of cement to grow a container garden. Many fruits, vegetables, and herbs can be grown in containers. Yes, it's a little more work initially than running to the grocery store to pick up some basil or jalapeños, but it's worth it. It enables you to grow your plants organically, which gives you peace of mind. I also promise you that your herbs and produce will taste better and be healthier for you than anything you can buy in the store.

If you get your kiddos to help you pick out the seeds and plant them, guess what? They'll want to eat the fruits, veggies, and herbs, too! I know it sounds too good to be true, but it really works. One caveat is that you need to buy organic seeds to ensure that they aren't genetically modified, which brings me to my next argument for organic food.

GMO

Even if you don't know what "genetically modified organism" or "GMO" means, I'm sure you've heard of it or seen it on a label. When we're talking about food, "GMO" means the seeds have been genetically engineered to alter the crop in a way that makes it resistant to pests and/or produces food in a way that's more tasty and convenient. The problem with GMO items is that we don't know the long-term effects of manipulating what God gave us and putting it into our bodies.

Many industrialized countries have bans on GMO products or require labeling so that consumers can make informed decisions when purchasing food items. The United States doesn't require labeling of these items. In fact, the only way the average consumer knows whether or not a food is GMO is by the label "Non-GMO Project Verified" or "Certified Organic." Other than that, it's anyone's guess. It's likely that the majority of the food you're feeding your family has been genetically modified, such as corn (high-fructose corn syrup, corn syrup, corn starch), soy, canola, and wheat items found in many processed foods, unless you're buying food with those non-GMO or certified organic labels. This brings me to my next point. It's a good one too so keep reading!

Organic Food in a Box

When buying food that comes in a package, you never know what kind of science experiment you might find. What I mean by this is simply that many of the ingredients are chemical compounds you can't pronounce, never mind find in nature (find me some sodium benzoate in your backyard, I dare you). For this reason, buying organic items may be a better option. Please don't misunderstand me; real and whole foods are the best tools to build strong, healthy bodies, but if you're going to buy something in a box, organic should be a consideration. The reason for this is that you won't find high-fructose corn syrup or GMO products in the box. Most of the time, the ingredients will be familiar and easy for you to pronounce.

Organic food is held to a higher standard, and I'm so thankful for that. Yes, you pay more, but that's because organic farmers have to pay to verify that their food is organic, and they make very little profit for the time they spend honoring your body and this planet. Meanwhile, food companies can pick up cheap GMO ingredients (which receive government funding, therefore making them a lot cheaper than organic foods) for their products, put almost anything in a box, call it food, and turn a large profit without having to prove its worthiness to be called food.

Cost Comparison

The argument against organic food always falls back on the cost. While I won't argue that in general it costs more, I will argue that if it can fit in your budget, it's worth every penny. And remember, you get what you pay for! So in honor of this argument, I thought I would go to a local grocery store and see what the difference in cost was in organic and conventional items.

I compared prices of common food staples and below I've listed the prices for comparison:

	Conventional	Organic
Gala apples:	$1.99/lb	$1.99/lb
Yams:	$1.49/lb	$2.99/lb
Mushrooms:	$1.99/ 8oz	$2.49/ 8 oz
Microwave popcorn:	$2.99/ 8 oz	$2.99/ 8 oz
Ketchup:	$1.49/ 20 oz	$1.99/ 20 oz
Brown rice:	$1.59/lb	$4.99/lb
Pasta sauce:	$2.00/ 24 oz	$2.50/ 25 oz
Sugar:	$1.59/ 32 oz	$3.69/ 32 oz
Peanut Butter	$3.99/ jar	$6.79/ jar
Milk	$2.99/ gallon	$5.29/ gallon

As you can see the organic prices vary from no difference, fifty cents more, and all the way up to more than twice as much as the conventional items. Did you know that you could get organic items for the same price as conventional? I'm willing to bet that most people don't know this and therefore don't even give organic items a glance.

That's the monetary cost. Let's talk about less tangible costs. Let's consider your family's health. How important is it to you to avoid cancer? How about for your kids or spouse? I imagine if you're reading this book, you care very much about your family's health.

The cancer risk has been steadily increasing over the past century. Why? Because our environment has become loaded with toxins. This means the air we breath, the water we drink, the food we eat, and pretty much every manmade material or device we come into contact with on a daily basis. We are literally poisoning ourselves sick.

Did you know that you have a 1 in 3 risk of getting cancer in your lifetime as a woman (1 in 2 risk for men), according to cancer.org? Did you also know that food can help you fight cancer? Specifically nutrient dense foods such as fruits and vegetables are helpful in fighting off cancer cells. I'm no expert and I'm certainly not a cancer doctor but it makes sense to me that if you're trying to heal your body, the best way to do that is to avoid adding more toxins into it. For that reason, organic is most beneficial. I say cut out the middle-man entirely, start eating lots of organic foods (especially produce), and avoid cancer all-together!

CHAPTER 7

Dining-Out Tips

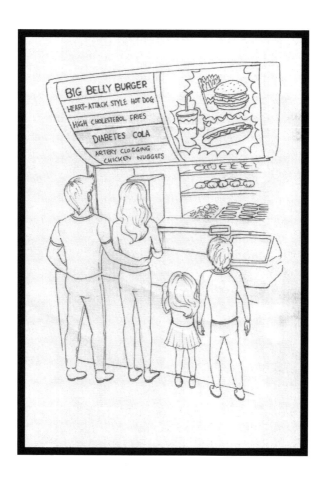

In an ideal world, we would all have time to be June Cleaver and have a delicious and nutritious dinner on the table promptly at 6:00 p.m. We don't live in an ideal world, and we certainly don't live in the world June Cleaver did. Life has sped up immeasurably since that era. Now most women work outside the home, and those who don't are breakneck busy with other obligations and pursuits. Sometimes eating out is the fastest and most convenient option. Sometimes you just need a night off from cooking. Sometimes you're simply craving the green curry from the local Thai restaurant and nothing else will do. I get it.

Because we live in the real world and not the ideal world, I thought I'd give you some tips to help you eat out without compromising your health or your waistline. These are tips I give to my clients and what I used when I lost thirty pounds, so they are tried and true. The key to successful eating outside of your home is planning ahead, knowing how to navigate social events, choosing healthier restaurants, eating only until you're full, and sharing your entrée or dessert. Simple and effective. Let's get started!

Planning Ahead

The key to successful dining out is planning ahead. I know you're thinking *If I had time to plan ahead, I'd be eating at home.* That is a valid point, but this planning requires only a three- to five minute Internet search for the nutrition facts of the restaurant you plan to attend. All large chain restaurants are required to provide this information. It becomes slightly more difficult if you're visiting a local, hole-in-the-wall restaurant, but I will help you navigate that as well.

Many restaurants have a "healthy eating" section of the menu or some way to denote the healthier choices. Some don't. That's okay too. Take a look at the menu that contains the nutrition information and make your choice based on the healthfulness of the dish (look for high fiber and protein and low cholesterol, saturated fat, sugar, and sodium). It may be difficult to find dishes that suit all of your dietary needs, just pick the one that fulfills most or the most important needs (example: the amount of sugar if you're a diabetic). Trust me, deciding what to order before you show up at the restaurant will increase the likelihood that you make a healthy choice.

You know how it is when you get to the restaurant and you're bombarded by amazing smells and everything on the menu sounds so delicious. Next thing you know, your stomach is speaking for your brain and you've ordered the double cheeseburger with curly fries and a chocolate shake. This especially happens when you can't plan ahead because you're at a social event and don't have prior access to a menu detailing the nutrition information of each item. No fear, I've got tips to help you with that too.

Navigating Social Events

Navigating social events can be tricky. Human beings seem to get into the mindset that calories consumed in groups don't count. Sadly, it doesn't work this way. But take heart, there are ways to enjoy yourself at events without hindering all your strides toward healthy eating.

A great trick I use is to have something to eat before I leave for the event. I'll have something small, such as vegetable soup, a salad, or a handful of nuts, to keep me from showing up at the party ravenous. I know many people "save up" their calories from earlier in the day to "spend" at the party. Don't do this! Your body uses only 300 to 400 calories at a time. Anything you eat above that will likely be stored as fat (especially if it's loaded with added sugars or refined carbohydrates).

Upon arrival, your host might offer you a drink. I suggest that you start off with water. Avoid soda. It's loaded with empty calories, and you're likely to have too much. After you've had water, if you'd like a fruity beverage with an umbrella, feel free. Enjoy one drink. Any drink you want, but just one! Then go back to drinking water.

Once you're ready to eat, fill up half of your plate with veggies. This will help ensure that you get lots of nutrition without all the calories and saturated fat. It also will help you fill your tummy and keep you from indulging in less healthy options.

After you fill your plate, walk away from the food. Don't hang out near the buffet; it's too tempting. How many times have you mindlessly eaten something at a party because it was sitting in front of you? You know this has happened when you're thinking back and you have no idea how many chips or buffalo wings you ate while you were chatting with Aunt Jo-Jo.

Some events involve sit-down meals that don't allow you the choice of what goes on your plate. In this case, refer to my tips for dine-in restaurants in the next section. Those tips will help you navigate this sticky situation, too.

If possible, sit down and enjoy your food. Take a good look at it. Say a little prayer or thank the host for the spread. Being mindful of the fact that you're eating and about what you're putting in your body will make the meal a satisfying experience.

Once you've finished your tasty meal, wait thirty minutes before going back for seconds or dessert. This will give your stomach time to tell your brain whether or not you've had enough to eat. Most of the time, it will tell you to stop. If the dessert looks too good to pass up, ask your host for a doggie bag to take a piece home with you. Trust me, he won't be offended.

Healthy-Option Restaurants

There are restaurants out there that make impromptu dining out a breeze because the majority of their items are on the healthy side. Restaurants that specialize in soup, salads, and sandwiches are a good bet. Look for restaurants that have well-appointed salad bars or nutrition-packed salads (more than just lettuce, tomato, and onion on them). Panera and Jason's Deli are good choices. Another restaurant that can prepare healthful options is Chipotle. These restaurants not only give you healthful options; they also provide food that has been selected because of the quality, such as antibiotic-free chicken (trust me, this matters). In a pinch, Subway will work, too. It has more chains available across the United States than the other restaurants listed.

Remember, though, just because you're in a healthy restaurant doesn't mean all of the items on the menu are good for you. When choosing soup, think *clear broth, meat, and veggies*. When choosing sandwiches, think *lean meat with lots of veggies on whole-grain bread* (preferably with noticeable grains and seeds in and on the bread). When choosing a salad or the salad bar, stay away from potato and macaroni salads, cheese, croutons, tortilla chips, and creamy dressings. If God made it, eat it. The more veggies you pile on your plate, the better. Think in terms of color. The more colorful the food you eat, the more nutrients it contains.

Fast Food

In a fast-food restaurant, salad is hands down your healthiest option. Order it with grilled chicken to add protein, and have them make it without cheese, bacon, or croutons. Also be mindful of the dressing you put on top. All fast-food chains have a low-calorie dressing; don't be afraid to ask for it. Don't feel like a salad? Order a grilled chicken sandwich without the bun. Most restaurants are happy to wrap it in lettuce instead. Or, if it's available, order a grilled chicken wrap without cheese or creamy condiments.

For your kiddos, I recommend either the smallest size (four pieces rather than six) of chunked and formed chicken product (um, I mean chicken nuggets) or a hamburger with whatever fruit side they offer. I recommend water to drink for your kiddos, but if that just won't do, then get either milk or juice. *Never, ever* get your kids (or yourself) diet soda. The harm you will do by allowing those chemicals into their precious little bodies is not worth the calories and sugar you will save by choosing diet over regular soda!

Dine-In Restaurants

Ah, fine dining, or maybe not. Either way, here are some tips to help you avoid consuming an entire day's worth of calories, fat, sodium, and cholesterol in one meal. First, eighty-six the bread basket or tortilla chips that the waiter so graciously brings to fill out your waistline, um, I mean your stomach. You know that if it's sitting there in front of you while you wait for your food, you'll eat it. Even if you vow to God, before you enter the restaurant, that you won't touch it, you will.

Next, order a garden salad or clear-broth vegetable soup to begin your meal. Make sure the salad contains only vegetables. Get your dressing on the side so that you control the amount. Opt for vinaigrettes and stay far away from creamy dressings such as ranch, Caesar, or creamy Italian. This will ensure that you get your veggies in and keep you from overeating your entrée.

Now, on to the entrée. Always ask the waiter to bring a takeout box with your meal, unless you plan to share your entrée with a friend or loved one. This way you can box up what you don't eat immediately when you're full or be proactive and box up half the meal before the fork touches your lips. I don't know about you, but if my plate of delicious food is still in front of me when I'm full, I will pick off of it until it's empty. This will save you calories and that ridiculously, uncomfortable full feeling you get after overindulging.

If you'd like to keep your entrée to yourself or you're really hungry, here are a few suggestions to aid your healthful choices:

1. Choose meat that's grilled or baked, never fried.
2. Skip added sauces or gravy.
3. Avoid items on the menu that are described as braised, creamed, au gratin, scalloped, smothered, stuffed, sautéed, or any of the various code words for fried, including crispy, battered, breaded, golden, or tempura.

Whenever possible, choose brown rice instead of pasta or potatoes, and when that's not an option, replace your starchy side with a vegetable or have a plain baked potato. Rethink your plate! Instead of one serving each of meat, starch, and vegetables, have a serving of meat and two vegetables. If you're vegan or vegetarian, have a starch and two vegetables. One caveat is that your veggies must be naked.

DINING-OUT TIPS

Herbs and spices are permissible and even recommended. Other than that, no butter, no oil, no cheese. No fun, right? Wrong. Once you stop burying your food in heaps of dairy and fat, you actually get to enjoy the real flavor, and I'm here to tell you—it's enjoyable!

One final tip for you when eating out: Don't drink your calories! You've gone to all this trouble to ensure that you're on the right track. Don't blow it with three refills of Coke because they're free and unlimited. If you feel the need to partake in a sweetened drink or alcoholic beverage, by all means enjoy. The key is to enjoy—only one—and then switch to drinking water for the rest of the meal.

Now, tips for feeding your kiddos. Have you ever looked at the kids' menu and thought, *Are you kidding me?* No? Maybe that's just me. Why are we feeding our children meals that are loaded with saturated fat, cholesterol, sodium, and sugar? Oh, that's right. It's because that's what *we're* eating. My suggestion for you is to forgo the kid's meal altogether. Order them something off the regular menu but ask for a half portion or share your meal with them. Kids will be resistant to this at first, but when they see you're sticking to your decision (this requires that you actually stick to it and not give in), they will give up the battle.

Trust me, I've recently gone through this with my kiddos, who are fourteen and nine years old and not particularly thrilled to have their mom become a vegan. There was pushback, but I didn't give in, and it didn't last long. Are they vegans? No, because that's a very personal decision. Do they eat less meat and dairy and more fruits, vegetables, legumes, and whole grains as a result of my veganism? Absolutely. Do they love it? Nope! Do they deal with it? Yup! I'm not giving you this advice because I'm perfect (not even close). I'm giving you this advice because I've been where you are, and I had to figure out the hard way how to get to where I am, which is the best health of my life at thirty-six years old. I don't want you to have to take the long road there and suffer the consequences of ill health along the way.

Dessert

Life is too short to give up dessert! Especially molten-chocolate cake, hot-fudge brownie sundaes, or tiramisu. With that said, you don't need dessert every day. Dessert should be a treat; something you have occasionally. When you do have dessert, share it! Trust me, there will be more than enough calories and sugar to go around (and around). Nothing is better than ending the day sharing a dessert and a good laugh with your family. Unless, of course, you're fighting over the last bite or the biggest bite, but I digress (you know you've been there). If that sounds like your family, I suggest you look for small, individual desserts. Order the smallest cup of ice cream. No one needs anything bigger than the kid's-size cup! The size doesn't matter. Focus on the experience and enjoy every bite. Make it worth the calories and sugar!

Enjoy it immensely and ignore guilt. Getting and staying healthy isn't about depriving yourself of delicious foods; it's about finding balance. Eat dessert but eat it less often than fruits, vegetables, beans, healthful meats, nuts, seeds, and whole grains. Strive for 80 percent healthy foods and 20 percent indulgent foods. Once you achieve this balance you can step off the diet roller coaster and enjoy true freedom.

Conclusion

It is my sincerest hope that you use the information contained in this book to improve the lives of you and your family. Making the choice and taking action to feed your family healthy food will have a profound impact on their physical and mental well being. Making the choice and taking action to take care of yourself will have an equally profound effect. Don't ever underestimate the importance of a well taken care of momma! You take care of everyone else; you deserve the same respect. Don't ever feel guilty for investing some of your time and energy in you.

Motherhood is the most beautiful and exhausting experience in life. You're blessed with the care-taking and future productivity training of human beings. That's a big deal! Consider yourself the CEO of a Fortune 500 company, who also happens to be the janitor, security guard, cleaning crew, food service coordinator, and accountant; I could go on but you get the picture. It's not a glamorous job. You work twenty-four hours a day, seven days a week, and 365-366 days a year. Find me one CEO who works those hours! You won't. Find me one CEO who doesn't get weekends off and vacation days. You won't find that either. There is a good reason for this. No one can be at peak performance if they don't take time for themselves.

As the mom, you're steering the bus. You have the opportunity to change your family's quality of life with the information you learned in the pages of this book. Consider your genes to be more like suggestions. Your environment (how you live and what you eat) influences whether or not genes express themselves. What I'm saying is that your relatives' fate, even your parents' fate, doesn't belong to you! Make the decision right now to make health a priority in your home and you will reap the benefits for years and generations to come.

Use this book as the first weapon in your arsenal to combat ill health caused by poor diet. I have provided you with lots of helpful information but it's only helpful if you actually put it to use. To make that easier, I have added a couple handy pull out pages. These pages are to be torn out and placed in your purse or wallet for quick reference when you're grocery shopping. I don't expect you to remember every juicy nugget of information I provide you with. I do expect you to use what's most important to you to improve the health and wellness of your family. These pages will make that easier for you.

CONCLUSION

Now that you know more than the average person about health and how to increase it, go forth, and spread your knowledge. Please share this information with everyone you know. Recommend this book to your friends and family who want to eat better but struggle with the constant barrage of misinformation provided by the media. I promise, they'll thank you for it.

One last thing, please read through until the end of the book. You will find out how you can work with me, individually or in groups, and solicit my employment for articles or speaking endeavors. I have also listed books and movies that have helped me along my journey, which you might find enlightening. Finally, you'll find the tear-out quick reference guides I added to help you make healthful choices for your family when you're out at the grocery store wrestling up dinner.

Need More Personalized Attention to Reach Your Goals? I'd be happy to help!

You're probably wondering *What the heck is a health coach?* A couple of years ago, I would've shrugged my shoulders and answered an honest *dunno!* Of course, now that I am one, I'd be more than happy to answer that question for you because health coaches are the future of wellness care. We are the answer to the current "sick care" crisis in the United States and around the globe.

As a health coach I work with busy moms who want to lose weight, increase energy, and feed their families healthy food in a hurry. I'm the Busy Mom's Health Coach. I've done all the research and given up years of my time educating myself on everything that's involved with health (physical, emotional & spiritual) and nutrition, so that you don't have to. After all, as a busy mom, you don't have that kind of time!

Together we formulate a wellness plan for you that will enhance your life in numerous ways. You see, we focus on *food* as one of the ways of nourishing your body with the understanding that it's not the only way and in most cases, not the most important form of nourishment you need in your life. As a woman you require nourishment from spirituality, relationships, career, and physical activity, in addition to good, old-fashioned food.

Regardless of your starting point on the journey to wellness you will receive individualized attention from me from the beginning to the end of your journey. You don't have to do this alone. I'm here to help and I promise, with time and effort on your part, you will achieve and may even surpass your initial goals.

I've been where you are. I know the feelings of frustration and confusion that surround health. One week coffee is the devil and the next it's a super food (and what the heck is a *super food* anyway?). Are eggs bad? Is fat the enemy? Do carbs make me gain weight or give me energy? How much protein is enough? What are antioxidants and why do I need them? How do I get little Melissa to eat her broccoli? Can I introduce new foods without my family resisting? How do I help my kids lose weight without making them self-conscious? You don't have to have all the answers or spend days searching for them. I've done the research for you!

Not only have I done the research but I've also been trained by the best of the best at the Institute for Integrative Nutrition. Guest lecturers include Dr. Andrew Weil; Marion Nestle, Ph.D; Dr. Mark Hyman (one of my faves!); Dr. Barry Sears; Dr. Frank Lipman; and so many more amazing people who are the subject-matter experts in their fields. I could fill a whole chapter with their names! Rest assured, you're in good hands.

What I have to offer you is knowledge interweaved with love, understanding, and a listening ear. I am your cheerleader and your drill sergeant. I'm your health guru and your favorite confidante. I am the person with the tools you need to succeed. Partner with me and make the change you've been aching to make for years. Don't hesitate! Contact me now for your complimentary health history consultation.

If you're still hesitant, read this testimonial from a busy momma who participated in one of my sugar detox groups:

Yesterday I completed my 10-Day Sugar Detox. I thought I would say something about it because I am pretty "average American" on the way I eat/live and I am pretty open about most things. We have pizza night, I drink soda, I eat fast food sometimes when I am out, I eat meat, I love to bake and cook, I don't workout as often as I should, I have a sweet tooth, and actually EAT food, but also care about getting to a healthy weight and living to see my kids grow up. I learned a lot about "hidden sugars" through this process, and how to adjust my meals so I wouldn't starve to death! That being said, **I lost a total of 7.5lbs, 3 inches off my waist, and**

busted through my weight loss plateau that has plagued me for the last month, surpassing the 40lb mark putting my total loss to date at 42 pounds. I'm not gonna lie, it was tough, but I feel like I have a better grasp on the nutrition side of weight loss. I would suggest something like this to anyone who feels like they have sort of "gone off the rails" a bit, say after the holiday, and wants to get back on track. Thank you Jennifer for having me in your group and teaching me some valuable lessons.

-Megan N., mom of two

Another great testimonial from a health coaching client:

Before I met Jennifer I was overweight, had constant back pain, trouble sleeping and was perpetually tired. Shortly after I met Jennifer I watched her transform her life and her body and I realized I wanted to do the same thing for myself. With her help ***I was able to lose 15 pounds in 3 months and have kept it off for over a year!*** Her constant encouragement and sincere desire to help me be better is what made me successful. She provided me with information on nutrition, fitness, and motivated me to make the changes I had wanted for so long. Now I am happy to say that I am pain free, sleep well at night, and have constant energy all day! The things I have learned from Jennifer will stick with me all my life. I am a better person because of her.
-Karen C., mom of four

NEED MORE PERSONALIZED ATTENTION...

To connect with me and receive my services head to my website to:

-sign up for my monthly newsletter and/or blog to get great tips and tricks for increasing health and harmony in your life.

-learn more about my current workshops, events, and speaking engagements.

-sign up for a complimentary health history consultation.

-learn more about me and what services I have to offer.

Send me an email to:

-hire me to speak at your event.

-employ me to write an article for your publication.

-learn more about my experience with the Institute for Integrative Nutrition, ask questions to see if it's a good fit for you, and receive a tuition discount.

Connect with me:

Website: jenniferbeverage.com
Website: jennifer-beverage.healthcoach.
integrativenutrition.com
Facebook: facebook.com/thebusymomshealthcoach
Email: jenniferbeveragehealthcoach@gmail.com

Recommended for Further Enlightenment:

Everything I recommend in this section has had a personal impact on me and it is my hope that the information contained in these books and videos speaks to you, as well.

Books:
21 Days to Master Success and Inner Peace by Dr. Wayne Dyer

Forget Fitting In: Your Path to Health and Happiness by Fitting Out by Jen Viano

Integrative Nutrition: Feed Your Hunger for Health & Happiness by Joshua Rosenthal

PUSH: 30 Days to Turbocharged Habits, a Bangin' Body, and the Life You Deserve! by Chalene Johnson

Raising Fit Kids in a Fat World by Judy Halliday, R.N. & Joani Jack, M.D.

The Compound Effect by Darren Hardy

Videos:
Fat, Sick and Nearly Dead

Fed Up

Forks Over Knives

Food Inc.

Food Matters

Vegucated

Tear-Out Guides for Quick Reference

Because this book is filled with lots of helpful tid bits of information, too many to immediately commit to memory, I thought you might find a couple quick reference guides useful. Simply tear out the pages, place them in your purse, wallet, or diaper bag and bring them with you when you venture out to do your grocery shopping.

The Dirty Dozen & The Clean Fifteen

That title sounds more like a mob movie than a recommendation for produce! In case you've forgotten, the *dirty dozen* refers to the twelve items of produce most contaminated with pesticides and the *clean fifteen* refers to the items of produce that are least contaminated with pesticides. Therefore, it is recommended that you purchase the dirty dozen organically grown, while the clean fifteen you can purchase conventionally grown. Find more in depth information about this at ewg.org.

The Dirty Dozen	The Clean Fifteen
1. Apples	1. Avocados
2. Strawberries	2. Sweet Corn
3. Grapes	3. Pineapple
4. Celery	4. Cabbage
5. Peaches	5. Sweet Peas (frozen)
6. Spinach	6. Onions
7. Sweet Bell Peppers	7. Asparagus
8. Nectarines (imported)	8. Mangoes
9. Cucumbers	9. Papayas
10. Cherry Tomatoes	10. Kiwi
11. Snap Peas (imported)	11. Eggplant
12. Potatoes	12. Grapefruit

(Clean 15 continued)
13. Cantaloupe
14. Cauliflower
15. Sweet Potatoes

Helpful Quick Reference Shopping Tips

1. Remember to shop mainly in the outer aisles where the real, whole foods are located. These foods include meat, fruits, vegetables, eggs, dairy, nuts and seeds. For whole grains, venture into the center aisles.
2. When purchasing boxed or bagged items choose items with 3-5 ingredients that you can actually pronounce. Also consider organic due to the higher quality ingredients.
3. Better yet, purchase natural items that don't have labels because they contain only the item God made for you to consume.
4. If you feel the need to purchase a packaged item that doesn't fit in with the other suggestions but you really, really want to buy it, try to avoid the following additives and/or preservatives (Ch. 5):
   -artificial coloring   -sodium benzoate
   -high fructose corn syrup   -trans fat
   -monosodium glutamate   -aspartame
   -sodium nitrate
5. Remember to avoid the common traps (Ch. 4):
   -coupon trap   -endcap trap
   -sample trap   -hunger trap
   -flyer trap   -superstore trap

6. Don't forget to stick to your list. This will help you avoid buying items you didn't intend to purchase, keep you from falling victim to the common traps, and keep your budget in check. Never, ever set foot in the grocery store without a list. Not even if you're only buying milk! Your list ensures you buy only what you need.

Made in the USA
San Bernardino, CA
13 April 2015